Manel Boudokhane
Hiba Bettaieb
Ons Hamdi

Static foot disorders and low back pain: what's the hidden link?

Manel Boudokhane
Hiba Bettaieb
Ons Hamdi

Static foot disorders and low back pain: what's the hidden link?

ScienciaScripts

Imprint

Any brand names and product names mentioned in this book are subject to trademark, brand or patent protection and are trademarks or registered trademarks of their respective holders. The use of brand names, product names, common names, trade names, product descriptions etc. even without a particular marking in this work is in no way to be construed to mean that such names may be regarded as unrestricted in respect of trademark and brand protection legislation and could thus be used by anyone.

Cover image: www.ingimage.com

This book is a translation from the original published under ISBN 978-620-6-72482-7.

Publisher:
Sciencia Scripts
is a trademark of
Dodo Books Indian Ocean Ltd. and OmniScriptum S.R.L publishing group

120 High Road, East Finchley, London, N2 9ED, United Kingdom
Str. Armeneasca 28/1, office 1, Chisinau MD-2012, Republic of Moldova, Europe
Printed at: see last page
ISBN: 978-620-8-27670-6

TABLE OF CONTENTS

INTRODUCTION

Common low back pain is one of the most common disorders, affecting up to 80% of the general population at some point in their lives [1]. The first episode can occur at a young age, from the twenties onwards, but the prevalence of this condition is higher in older subjects [2]. Several interrelated risk factors contribute to the development of common low back pain, including age, gender, obesity, occupation and psychosocial factors [2]. In addition to these well-established risk factors, the presence of foot static disorders has been incriminated in the predisposition to low back pain [3,4]. Indeed, abnormal posture and/or function of the feet can modify the stresses exerted on the peri-vertebral muscles and soft tissues [5]. It has been suggested that individuals with mechanical low back pain are more likely to have flat feet [6]. Although biomechanical and staturopostural changes in the lower limbs, including the feet, have been described by many authors, the relationship between foot statics disorders and common low back pain remains a matter of debate. A large retrospective study including 97,279 military personnel with moderate to severe flatfoot reported twice as much presence or history of mechanical low back pain compared to subjects with normal footbed [7]. However, other smaller-scale studies found no association between low back pain and foot statics disorders [6,8]. Despite this difference of opinion, the association between these two entities is biomechanically and physiologically plausible. It has been shown that variation in the length of the the internal longitudinal arch influenced the amplitude of acceleration during running at spinal level [9], as did the position of the feet, which modified pelvic alignment [3,10,11] and the electromyographic activity of the erector and gluteal muscles during walking [12]. In addition, several other studies have shown the effect of prescribing corrective foot orthoses in reducing the intensity of low back pain [13,14]. The aim of this study was to evaluate the association between foot statics disorders and common low back pain.

PATIENTS AND METHODS

1. Characteristics of the study :

This was a descriptive, comparative, cross-sectional, single-centre study involving two groups of patients:

❖ Group 1: "Study group > comprising 20 patients with common low back pain associated with foot static disorders. All patients in this group underwent lumbar spine radiography.

❖ Group 2: "Control group > comprising 20 patients with foot statics problems, matched to the group by age and gender.

These patients were included over a consecutive period from January to June 2021 during a rheumatology consultation at the Internal Security Forces Hospital in La Marsa.

2. Inclusion criteria :

2.1. Study group :

-Patients with common low back pain of at least six months' duration.

-Patients over 18 years of age.

-Patients who agreed to take part in the study.

2.2. Control group :

-Patients over 18 years of age.

-Patients who agreed to take part in the study.

3. Non-inclusion criteria :

3.1. Study group :

-Pregnant patients.

Patients who, in addition to common low back pain, have another non-mechanical pathology affecting the spine.

-Any disease affecting the cognition and the abilitiescomprehension.

-Patients undergoing spinal and/or foot surgery.

3.2. Control group :

-Any disease affecting the cognition and the abilities comprehension.

-Foot surgery patients.

4. Exclusion criteria :

4.1. Study group :

Patients with poor-quality X-rays of the lumbar spine, including those of small size.

-Patients with sequelae of foot deformities such as clubfoot, talus foot or convex foot.

4.2. Control group :

-Any pathology of the lower limbs that may interfere with foot statics (length asymmetry of the lower limbs, fracture of the lower limbs, foot surgery).

-Patients with sequelae of foot deformities such as clubfoot, talus foot or convex foot.

5. Data collection (Appendix 1) :

A form was drawn up to record data from the interview and clinical examination. A questionnaire assessing the functional impact of low back pain (for the study group) was completed by the examiner.

5.1. Patient characteristics :

Questioning a allowed to collect the (study and control groups):

❖ Age.

❖ Sex.

❖ The profession.

❖ Where you live: urban or rural.

❖ Background.

❖ Taking part in sporting activities.

❖ Body mass index (BMI).

5.2. Clinical characteristics of common low back pain (study group) :

Duration of low back pain in years. The visual analogue scale (VAS) for low back pain.

Physical examination data :

► The presence of signs of spinal stiffness: finger-to-ground distance, Schbber index.

► The presence of a radicular syndrome (Lasègue, sonnette).

► Walking on the balls and heels of your feet.

► Examination of the hips.

► Knee statics.

► Neurological examination. Therapeutic modalities :

► The various treatments received by the patients were

Specified: analgesics according to WHO levels, non-steroidal anti-inflammatory drugs (NSAIDs) (how they are taken), muscle relaxants, antidepressants, pregabalin, physical treatment, epidural infiltration and acupuncture.

Assessment of functional impact :

► Functional Incapacity Evaluation Scale for Low Back Pain (EIFEL) questionnaire (appendix 2) [15]. The

The total score is calculated by adding up the number of boxes ticked for the 24 questions. The higher the total score, the greater the functional impact of the low back pain. Radiological assessment: This was based on a frontal and lateral X-ray of the lumbar spine. The images were interpreted by a rheumatologist qualified in osteoarticular imaging. Signs of disc disease, posterior inter-apophyseal osteoarthritis, a narrow lumbar canal or spondylolisthesis were identified.

5.3. Study of disorders of the statics (study and control groups) :

Interview data collected :

❖ A history of talalgia and/or metatarsalgia.

❖ The characteristics of the talalgia and/or current metatarsalgia: location, laterality and time of day.

❖ The presence of fitting difficulties.

❖ Wearing safety shoes or uniforms. Foot examination data:

▶ The type of feet: Egyptian, square or Greek.

▶ The presence of areas of hyper-pressure: hyperkeratosis (calluses) or corns.

▶ Skin disorders: onychodystrophy or intertrigo.

▶ The type of foot deformity (hallux valgus, hallux

rigidus, hammer toe, claw toe, quintus varus, supra or infra-adductus) as well as their reducibility.

▶ The presence of exquisite pain points and their locations.

▶ Ankle and foot joint range of motion.

▶ Neurological and vascular examination of the feet.

▶ Gait examination. Podoscopic examination:

▶ Footbed: normal, flat foot or hollow foot.

▶ The angle between the axis of the leg and the heel on a posterior view (physiological valgus, valgus or varus).

▶ The appearance of the calcaneus and Achilles tendon.

▶ The presence of a protrusion of the tubercle medial of the navicular bone.

Examination of footwear :

▶ Heel height in centimetres (cm).

▶ How the shoe closes.

▶ Areas of wear on the sole and/or heel.

▶ Examination of foot orthoses.

6. Statistical analysis :

The data were entered and analysed using Statistical Package for Social Sciences version 26 software.

6.1. Descriptive study :

We carried out a descriptive study, calculating absolute frequencies for qualitative variables, and means, standard deviations and extremums for quantitative variables.

6.2. Analytical study :

We also conducted an analytical study. To study the link between common low back pain and foot statics disorders, we used Student's t-test, taking the foot statics disorders group as the control group for the population suffering from common low back pain. In all statistical tests, the significance level was set at 0.05.

7. Bibliography :

We used the PubMed and Science direct electronic databases to select articles of interest using the following keywords: low back pain, flat foot, hollow foot, foot static disorders, and their English corollaries.

The search was completed by a manual search of the articles using the references of the most relevant studies.

a.Ethics :

Our patients were informed of the purpose of the study beforehand and consented to the use of their clinical and paraclinical data for this study.

9. Conflicts of interest :

We declare that we have no conflict of interest in relation to this work.

RESULTS

The 40 patients were divided between the two groups as follows:

▶ Study group: 20 patients with common low back pain and foot static disorders.

▶ Control group: 20 patients with foot statics problems.

1. Patient characteristics :

1.1. Age :

The mean age for the study group was 65.2 ± 11.5 years with a median of 43 years [20 to 79 years]. The mean age for the control group was 60.9 ± 8.6 years, with a median of 40 years [21 to 74 years]. The age distribution of patients in the two groups is summarised in Figure 1.

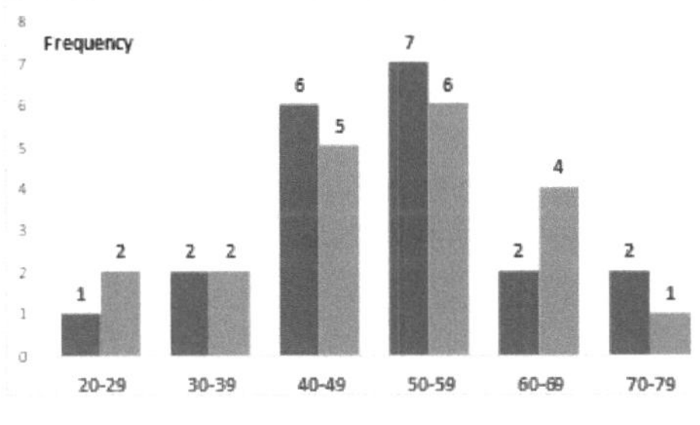

Figure 1: Breakdown of patients by age group.

1.2. Gender :

Our study included 13 female patients (65%) and seven male patients (35%) in each of the two groups. The sex ratio was 0.35.

1.3. Profession :

In both groups, the majority of patients were active. Forty-five per cent of patients were in heavy labour and 65% in office work. Fifteen percent of patients were retired.

1.4. Place of residence :

All the patients included in our study lived in an urban area.

1.5. Sporting activities :

Thirteen patients in the study group (65%) did not engage in any sporting activity. Seven patients practised several sporting activities. The sports activities practised were as follows: walking (7 patients), running (1 patient), swimming (3 patients), cycling (4 patients) and weight training (3 patients). In the control group, only five patients practised sport.

1.6. BMI :

For the study group, the mean BMI was 31.6 ± 6 kg/m^2 with extremes ranging from 19.9 to 43.1 kg/m^2 . For the control group, the average BMI was 30.2 ± 7.6 kg/m^2 with extremes ranging from 18 to 38.3 kg/m .^{2}

2. **Clinical characteristics of common low back pain (study group)**
:

2.1. **Duration and intensity of pain :**

The mean duration of low back pain was 14.6 ± 3 years, with extremes of 4 and 64 years. The mean duration of the current episode of low back pain was 64 days. The mean VAS for low back pain was 6.6 ± 1/10.

2.2. **Physical examination data :**

Spinal and radicular syndromes were noted in 80% and 70% of cases, respectively. Walking on heels was possible in all patients, whereas it was difficult on toes in 40% of patients. Examination of the hips was normal in all cases. An abnormality of knee statics was noted in 55% of patients, with genu varum and genu valgum in 7 and 4 patients respectively.

2.3. **Therapeutic methods :**

Treatment based on level I and II analgesics was prescribed in 70% and 30% of cases respectively. Half the patients were taking NSAIDs. NSAIDs were taken continuously in 80% of cases and on demand in 20%. The different treatment modalities are detailed in Table I.

Table I: The various therapeutic methods prescribed :

Treatment	Percentage (%)
Analgesic	100
NSAIDS	60
Muscle relaxant	30
Antidepressant	5
Pregabalin	10
Physical treatment	30
Epidural infiltration	30
Acupuncture	24

2.4. Functional impact :

The mean EIFEL score was 9.6 ± 2.1 with extremes between 0 and 11. Significant functional impairment with a score of 24/24 was noted in two patients (10%).

2.5. Radiological assessment :

X-rays of the lumbar spine showed abnormalities in 80% of cases. Figure 2 summarises the various abnormalities found on the X-rays.

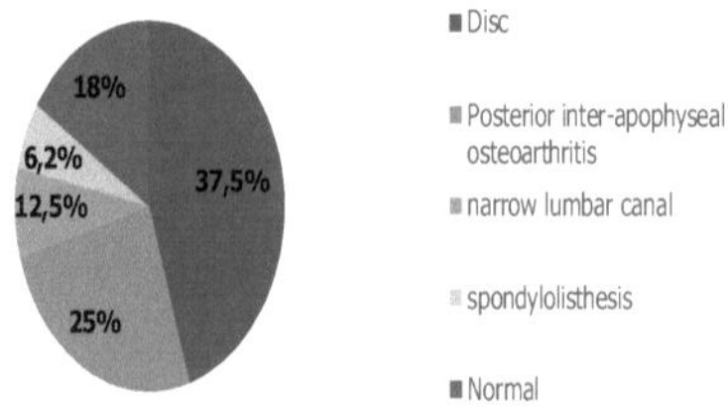

Figure 2: Radiographic abnormalities of the lumbar spine.

3. **Study of foot statics disorders :**

3.1. **Study group :**

3.1.1. **History :**

Talalgia was noted in 50% of cases (inferior 40%, posterior 30%, bipolar 30%). Twenty-five percent of patients had metatarsalgia. Talalgia and metatarsalgia were mechanical in all cases. Seven patients (35%) reported difficulty with footwear. Safety shoes or uniforms were worn in half of the cases. These were mainly the shoes worn by security officers (Brodequin high-top safety shoe).

3.1.2. **Data from the physical examination of the feet :**

Foot types were distributed as follows: Egyptian (55%), Greek (25%) and square (20%). Plantar hyperkeratosis was present in 75% of cases, with calluses in 65% and calluses in 55%. Twenty percent of patients had a horn. As regards skin disorders, onychodystrophy and intertrigo were present in 30% and 15% of cases, respectively. Sixty-five per cent of patients had foot deformities. The deformities were irreducible in half the cases. The different types of deformity are shown in Figure 3. Exquisite painful points on palpation were found in 30% of cases. Table II summarises the proportion of patients with limited range of motion in the ankle and foot joints. The neurological examination and gait study were within normal limits in all patients.

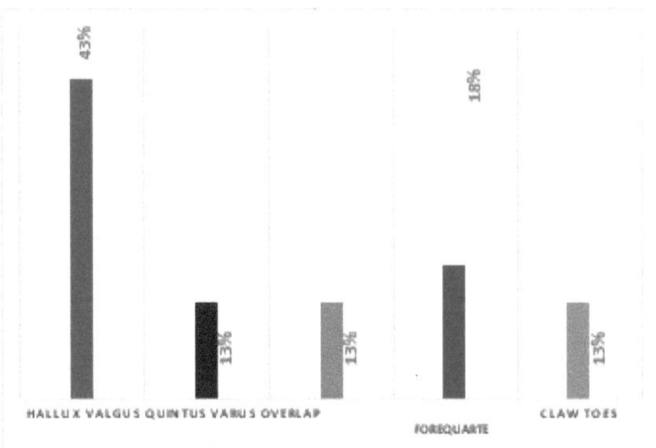

Figure 3: The different deformations of the feet in the study group.

Table II: Proportion of ankle and foot joint range of motion limitation in the study group :

Joint	Talo-crural	Subtalar	Chopart	Lisfranc	MTP*	IP
Limitation %	30	20	15	10	5	5

***MTP**: metatarsophalangeal ****IP**: interphalangeal

3.1.3. Data from the podoscopic examination :

An abnormal footbed was noted in all patients, with flat feet in 65% of cases and hollow feet in 35%. Figures 4 and 5 show the classification of flat and hollow feet, respectively. Valgus and varus of the hindfoot were present in 25% and 15% of cases, respectively. No patient had Achilles tendinopathy. Three patients (15%) had a protrusion of the medial tubercle of the navicular bone.

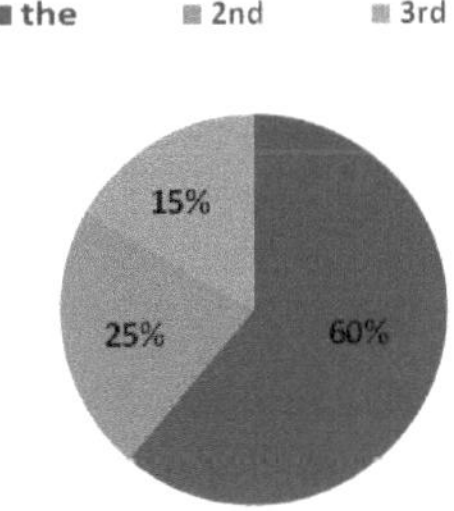

Figure 4: The study group's classification of flatfoot.

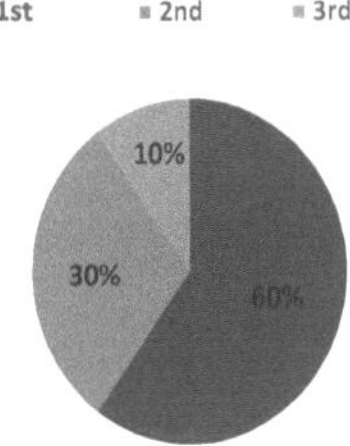

Figure 5: The study group's classification of the hollow foot.

3.1.4. Examination of footwear :

The average heel height was 3 cm. Shoes were fastened with laces in 80% of cases. Areas of sole wear were present in 45% of cases, distributed as follows: under the 1ère metatarsophalangeal (MTP) (56.2%), under the 2e 3e 4e MTP (50%), along the lateral edge of the sole (37.5%) and along the medial edge of the hallux (18.7%). None of the patients had plantar orthoses.

3.2. Control group :

3.2.1. History :

Talalgia was noted in 45% of cases (posterior 45%, inferior 33%, bipolar 22%). Thirty percent of patients had mechanical metatarsalgia. Difficulty with footwear was reported by nine patients. Wearing shoes or uniform parts were noted in 55% of cases.

3.2.2. Data from the physical examination of the feet :

The different types of feet were distributed as follows: Egyptian (60%), square (25%) and Greek (15%). Plantar hyperkeratosis was present in 60% of cases, with calluses in 45% and calluses in 65%. As for skin disorders, onychodystrophy and intertrigo were present in 25% and 10% of cases respectively. Seventy per cent of patients had foot deformities. The deformities were irreducible in 45% of cases. The type of foot deformity is shown in Figure 6. Exquisite painful points on palpation were found in 30% of cases. Table III summarises the proportion of patients with limited range of motion in the ankle and foot joints. The neurological examination and gait study were within normal limits in all patients.

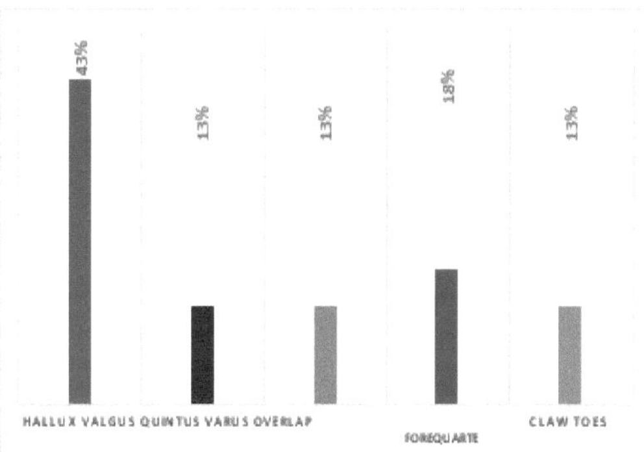

Figure 6: Foot deformities in the control group.

Table III: Proportion of ankle and foot joint range of motion limitation in the control group :

Joint	Talocrural e	Subtalar	Chopart	Lisfranc	MTP*	IP
Limitation %	31,2	18,7	25	12,5	6,2	6,2

***MTP**: metatarsophalangeal ****IP**: interphalangeal

3.2.3. Data from the podoscopic examination :

The different types of footbed were as follows: flat foot (70%) and hollow foot (30%). The classification of flat and hollow feet is shown in Figures 7 and 8, respectively. Valgus and varus of the hindfoot were present in 20% and 10% of cases, respectively. N o patient had a Achilles tendinopathy. Two patients had a protrusion of the medial tubercle of the navicular bone.

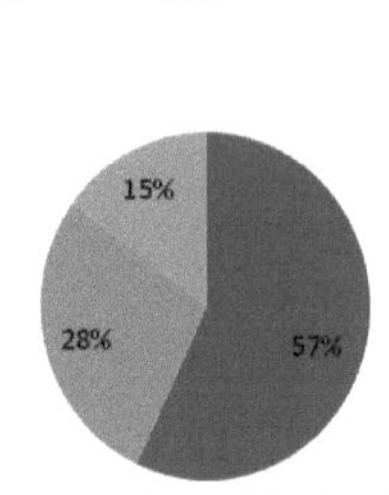

Figure 7: Classification of the flat foot in the control group.

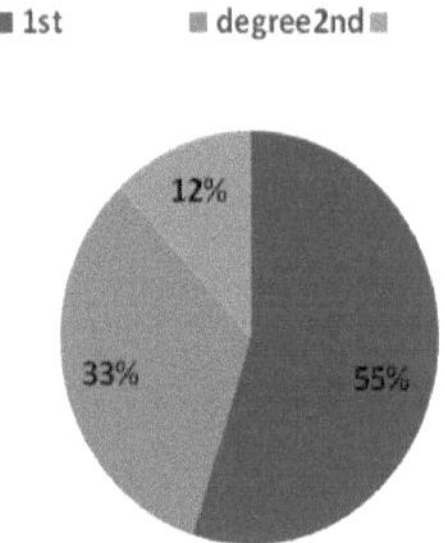

Figure a: Classification of the hollow foot in the control group.

3.2.4. Examination of footwear :

The average heel height was 3 cm. Shoes were fastened with laces in 85% of cases. Areas of sole wear were present in 40% of cases, distributed as follows: under the 1ère MTP (87.5%), under the 2e 3e 4e MTP (37.5%), the lateral edge of the sole (37.5%), under the head of the 1ère distal phalanx (25%) and along the medial edge of the hallux (12.5%). None of the patients had plantar orthoses.

4. **Study of the association between foot statics disorders and common low back pain :**

Common low back pain was significantly associated with foot statics disorders: toe deformity (p= 0.03), flat foot (p= 0.01), hollow foot (p= 0.01), hindfoot valgus (p= 0.00) and hindfoot varus (p= 0.00). The results of the comparison between the two groups of patients are summarised in Table III.

Table IV: Study of the association between foot statics disorders and common low back pain :

Variable	p
Talalgia	0,03
Metatarsalgia	0,30
Trophic disorders	0,07
Hyperkeratosis	0,05
Shoeing difficulties	0,21
Deformations	0,03
Flat foot	0,01
Hollow foot	0,01
Valgus of the hind foot	0,00
Varus of the hind foot	0,00
Protrusion of the medial tubercle of the navicular bone	0,09
Areas of wear on the shoe	0,13

DISCUSSION

Main results of the study :

Our study included two groups of patients: a study group comprising 20 patients suffering from common low back pain with foot statics disorders and a control group including 20 patients with foot statics problems without low back pain. Talalgia and metatarsalgia were present in 50% and 25% of cases in the study group, and 45% and 30% of cases in the control group, respectively. Hyperkeratosis was noted in 75% of the study group and 60% of the control group. Sixty-five per cent of patients in the study group and 70% in the control group had deformities of the feet and toes. Flat feet were present in 65% of patients in the study group and 70% in the control group. A hollow foot was noted in 35% of cases in the study group and 30% of cases in the control group. Valgus and varus of the hindfoot were present in 25% and 15% of cases in the study group, and 20% and 10% of cases in the control group, respectively. Forty-five per cent of the study group and 40% of the control group had areas of wear in their insoles. The results of the comparison between the two groups of patients concluded that the presence of foot statics disorders was significantly associated with common low back pain; talalgia (p= 0.03), hyperkeratosis (p= 0.05), presence of foot deformities (p= 0.03), flat foot (p=0.01), hollow foot (p= 0.01), valgus of the hind foot (p= 0.00) and varus of the hind foot (p= 0.00). In the light of these results, our study suggests the role of foot statics disorders as a risk factor for common low back pain. Orthotic treatment of these disorders of foot statics could play an important role in the management strategy for common low back pain.

Strengths and weaknesses of the study :

Our study presents many interesting points for several reasons:

■ The association between common low back pain and

Foot statics have been little studied in the literature [5- 8,16]. This is also the first study on a national scale.

■ We recruited patients randomly from a rheumatology consultation. Consequently, our

The sample is representative of patients attending a university hospital in Tunis.

■ According to recent consensus recommendations [17], the

The definition of patients with low back pain should also include questions on the duration and severity of the pain, which was the case in our study.

■ The inclusion of patients with pure mechanical low back pain, eliminating any underlying cause, shows that our sample is reliable for studying the causality of foot statics disorders in common low back pain.

Nevertheless, our study has a number of shortcomings:

■ The small number of patients included and the monocentric nature of the study may be considered as a weakness of the study. However, the number of doctors who are capable of carrying out a podiatry study in the various rheumatology departments remains limited.

Strengths and weaknesses of literature reviews :

Few studies have assessed the association between foot statics disorders and common low back pain [5- 8,16]. Among the strengths of the various studies in the literature, we should mention the Framingham study, which was based on the general population, and therefore its sample is more representative [5], unlike the other studies which were based on military [7] or clinical samples [6,8]. In addition, this study used an objective measurement of foot posture, which is a more objective method than visual assessment. It was also the first international study to incorporate measures of dynamic foot function.

However, these studies have a number of weaknesses. Firstly, these studies did not attempt to identify an underlying cause of low back pain, which could call into question the causality of foot static disorders [5,7]. In addition, in the Framingham study [5], the characteristics of low back pain were not specified (duration of course, severity of symptoms). It is therefore likely that the sample included patients with mild symptoms.

1. Patient characteristics :

❖ **Age:** In the literature, the mean age at inclusion was 64 years in the study by Framingham et al [5], and 31.23 years in the study by Framingham et al [6]. years for the mechanical low back pain group, and 28.82 years for the group without low back pain in the study by Brantingham et al [6]. The mean age at inclusion in our study was 65.2 ± 11.5 years for the study group and 60.9 ± 8.6 years for the control group.

❖ **Gender:** The predominance of women is one of the characteristics of osteoarthritis in general and low back pain in particular. mechanical in this case. The sex ratio in common low back pain in the various studies showed a predominance of women [5,6,8], which was the case in our study, where the sex ratio was 0.35.

❖ **Sports activities:** Seven patients in the study group and 5 patients in the control group took part in sports activities. sport. The majority of patients were sedentary. A sedentary lifestyle is often associated with excess weight and is a risk factor for mechanical low back pain.

❖ **BMI:** In studies which have examined the association between foot statics disorders and common low back pain, the mean BMI varied between 22 and 26 kg/m^2 [3,4,9,18]. The mean BMI in our study was 31.6 ± 6 kg/m^2 for the study group, and 30.2 ± 7.6 kg/m^2 for the control group, which was higher than the data in the literature.

2. Clinical characteristics of common low back pain (study group) :

In the literature, no other study on foot statics disorders with common low back pain has looked at clinical assessment of mechanical low back pain (physical examination, treatment modalities and imaging data).

2.1. Duration and intensity of pain :

The average duration of the current episode of low back pain was 64 days. In the literature, the mean duration ranged from 15.5 to 128 days [15,19]. The mean VAS for low back pain in Mendez's study ranged from 6.21 to 6.59/10 [13]. The mean VAS for low back pain in our study was 6.6/10, which is consistent with the literature.

2.2. Physical examination data :

To our knowledge, no other study in the literature has detailed the physical examination of patients with common low back pain associated with foot static disorders. The majority of our patients had signs of disco-radicular impingement. Examination of the hips was normal in all cases, ruling out any hip pathology that might have played a role in the genesis of mechanical low back pain. However, 55% of our patients had axially deviated knees. In the study by Kosashvili et al, there was a correlation between flatfoot and gonalgia [7], which implies an association between foot static disorders and knee pathologies.

2.3. Therapeutic methods :

A systematic review of European clinical practice guidelines on recommendations for the management of common low back pain emphasised the importance of physical treatment over NSAIDs, and even less so analgesics for pain. nociceptive [20]. In our study, all patients received symptomatic treatment: 100% drug treatment, 30% interventional treatment and 30% physical treatment.

2.4. Functional impact :

In the literature, the EIFEL score varied between 5.52 and 12 [21-23]. The functional impact of low back pain in our patients was moderate, with an average EIFEL score of 9.6. However, two patients had a score of 24, indicating severe functional impairment. The importance of the functional impact of low back pain may be increased by the presence of foot statics disorders.

2.5. Radiological assessment :

The most common radiographic abnormalities in common low back pain are disc impingement with or without a disc void and osteophytes [24] A systematic review of observational studies found that degenerative disc disease, defined by the presence of a pinched disc with osteophytosis and sclerosis, was the radiographic abnormality most associated with mechanical low back pain, with an odds ratio varying between 1.2 and 3.3 [25]. In our study, radiography of the lumbar spine was normal in only 20% of cases. The various abnormalities found were as follows: disc disease (37.5%), posterior inter-apophyseal osteoarthritis (25%), narrow lumbar canal (12.5%), and spondylolisthesis (6.2%).

3. Study of foot statics disorders :

3.1. Study group :

3.1.1. History :

Foot statics disorders often result in talalgia and/or metatarsalgia [26,27]. In our study, talalgia and metatarsalgia were frequent. Fifty percent and 25% of patients in the study group reported the presence of talalgia and metatarsalgia, respectively. These results were similar to those of the control group, with talalgia in 45% of cases and metatarsalgia in 35%.

3.1.2. Physical examination data :

Plantar hyperkeratosis was present in 75% of patients in the study group. In fact, architectural defects of the feet can lead to local skin overloads resulting in direct reactive hyperkeratosis linked to hyper-pressure or indirect hyperkeratosis linked to a vicious antalgic attitude [28]. Sixty-five percent of patients had foot deformities, half of which were irreducible. This rate is close to that of the control group, in which 70% of patients had foot deformities.

3.1.3. Data from the podoscopic examination :

In the study by Kosashvili et al [7], flatfoot was noted in 16.1% of the subjects included, 5% of whom had common low back pain. The severity of flatfoot was classified as follows: 74% mild, 21% moderate and 5% severe. In our study, 65% of patients with common low back pain had a flat foot. 35% had a hollow foot on podoscopic examination. The first degree was the most frequent stage in both types of abnormal footbed (60% in both cases).

3.1.4. Examination of footwear :

Areas of shoe wear were found in 45% of patients. These areas of wear reflect the age of the static foot problems, and their probable role as a factor favouring the persistence of mechanical low back pain that had been evolving for years. However, none of the patients wore a foot orthosis.

3.2. Control group :

3.2.1. History :

In the study by Khachat et al, most patients wore unsuitable footwear such as clogs and slippers [29]. In our study, nine patients reported difficulty with footwear. Uniform shoes were worn in 55% of cases.

3.2.2. Physical examination data :

In the literature, hyperkeratosis was found in 44% of cases [29]. In addition, examination of 100 feet revealed morphological disorders in 57 feet, such as hallux valgus (n= 31), claw toes (n= 22) and quintus varus (n= 4) [29]. Plantar hyperkeratosis was present in 60% of patients in the control group. The presence of deformities was more frequent in in the control group compared to the study group (70% versus 65%).

3.2.3. Data from the podoscopic examination :

In the study by Uhl et al [30], among 412 feet examined, a disorder of foot statics was found in 31% of cases, with a flat foot in 14.5% of cases and a hollow foot in 16.6% of cases. On podoscopic examination of 100 diabetic feet, a sunken foot was present in 26 cases and a hollow foot in 29 cases [29]. In our study, as in the study group, flat feet were more frequent than hollow feet (70% versus 30%). The first degree was also the most frequent stage, for both flatfoot (57%) and hollow foot (55%).

3.2.4. Examination of footwear :

In the study by Khachat et al, corrective foot orthoses were prescribed in 22% of cases [29]. In our study, the frequency of areas of shoe wear was similar between the two groups of patients (control group 40% versus study group 45%). No patients in the control group wore foot orthoses.

4. Study of the association between foot statics disorders and common low back pain :

Our study concluded that there was a significant association between foot statics disorders and common low back pain; talalgia (p= 0.03), hyperkeratosis (p= 0.05), foot deformities (p= 0.03), flat foot (p=0.01), hollow foot (p= 0.01), valgus of the hind foot (p= 0.00), and varus of the hind foot (p= 0.00). Our results were in line with those reported in the literature. Kosashvili et al found a higher prevalence of mechanical low back pain in patients with moderate to severe flatfoot (p= 0.001) [7]. These results also indicate that the prevalence of low back pain was proportional to the degree of severity of flat feet [7]. In a longitudinal cohort study with 14 years of follow-up including 2793 individuals, the authors found that patients with flat feet had a higher risk of having mechanical low back pain related to degenerative spinal pathology (42.3%, p<0.05) [16]. In the Framingham study, pronating foot was associated with mechanical low back pain [5]. Other studies in the literature have concluded that there is an association between flat foot [4,31,32] or hollow foot [7,33] and low back pain. The presence of low back pain in association with foot statics disorders is more frequent in women, which could be explained by the differences in alignment, degree of mobility and function of the pelvis and lower limbs between the two sexes [5]. Although foot orthoses represent a major expense for most of our patients, their therapeutic effects on mechanical low back pain have been attested to by several authors [13,14,34,35]. It is possible that plantar orthoses absorb shocks, thereby reducing stresses. on the spine, thereby improving mechanical low back pain [36]. Five randomised controlled trials have demonstrated an improvement in low back pain in patients who had plantar orthoses compared with those who had no orthoses [13,18,37,38]. It has also been shown that patients with flat feet may undergo reactive postural changes leading to compensatory imbalance between the spine and the lower limbs [39].

5. Recommendations:

In the light of the results of our study, we recommend : In the case of common low back pain, a systematic examination of the feet is essential, and should be carried out as early as the first consultation. Training in podiatry for rheumatologists, orthopaedists and family doctors is essential to familiarise them with this type of pathology and to ensure early diagnosis of foot statics disorders. In the case of any static foot disorder, it is essential to prescribe the appropriate treatment (orthotic, physical and/or surgical). In fact, treating foot statics disorders can also relieve common low back pain and should be part of the overall treatment.

6. Outlook:

However, larger-scale studies with prolonged follow-up seem necessary to confirm these results and thus enable a better assessment of the role of foot statics disorders in common low back pain, especially as the course of low back pain is intermittent and periodic. Further studies using objective measurements of foot statics would increase the strength of the results. Increasing the availability of podoscopes in rheumatology departments could improve the management of low back pain by detecting foot statics disorders at an early stage.

CONCLUSIONS

Low back pain is a common condition, affecting up to 80% of the general population of any age. Several risk factors are associated with the onset of low back pain. In addition to these well-established risk factors, the presence of foot static disorders has been incriminated in the predisposition to low back pain. Although biomechanical and staturopostural changes in the lower limbs have been described by numerous authors, the relationship between foot statics disorders and common low back pain remains a subject of debate. In this study, we assessed the association between foot statics disorders and common low back pain. We conducted a descriptive, cross-sectional, monocentric study including 40 patients divided into two groups: study group (common low back pain with foot statics disorders) and control group (foot statics disorders), followed up at the rheumatology consultation of the internal security forces hospital. The clinico-radiological and therapeutic characteristics of common low back pain were collected: length of time the pain had been present, pain intensity assessed by the EVA low back pain scale, signs of disco-radicular impingement, the various treatments prescribed (medicinal and non-medicinal), functional impact using the EIFEL questionnaire and abnormalities observed on lumbar spine radiography. A study of static disorders in the feet of patients in the two groups included the following data: the presence of areas of hyperkeratosis, deformities and their reducibility, and the presence of abnormalities in the lumbar spine. joint amplitudes. The podoscopic examination determined the type of footbed, the presence of valgus or varus of the hindfoot and the presence or absence of a protrusion of the medial tubercle of the navicular bone. The examination also included observation of the footwear. We then conducted an analytical study using Student's t-test to investigate the link between foot statics disorders and common low back pain. Talalgia and metatarsalgia were present in 50% and 25% of the study group, and 45% and 30% of the control group, respectively. Hyperkeratosis was noted in 75% of patients in the study group and 60% of patients in the control group. Sixty-five per cent of patients in the study group and 70% in the control group had foot deformities. Flat feet were present in 65% of patients in the study group and 70% in the control group. A hollow foot was noted in 35% of the study group and 30% of the control group. Valgus and varus of the hindfoot were present in 25% and 15% of the study group, and 20% and 10% of the control group, respectively. Forty-five per cent of the study group and 40% of the control group had areas of wear in their insoles. The results of the comparison between the two groups of patients concluded that there was an association between foot statics disorders and common low back pain; talalgia (p= 0.03), hyperkeratosis (p= 0.05), foot deformities (p= 0.03), flat foot (p=0.01), hollow foot (p= 0.01), hindfoot valgus (p= 0.00) and hindfoot varus (p= 0.00).In the light of these results, our study suggests the role of foot statics disorders as a risk factor. common low back pain. Therefore, in all cases of mechanical low back pain, the practitioner should carry out a podoscopic examination to detect foot statics disorders at an early stage, especially as orthotic treatment could play an important role in the therapeutic strategy for mechanical low back pain. In addition, larger-scale studies with prolonged follow-up seem necessary to confirm our results and allow a better assessment of the role of foot statics disorders in common low back pain.

REFERENCES

1. Lopez de Célis C, Barra M, Villar E. Correlaci6n entre dolor, discapacidad y rango de movilidad en pacientes con lumbalgia cr6nica - ScienceDirect. Fisioterapia. 2009;31:177-82.

2. Hoy D, Brooks P, Blyth F, Buchbinder R. The Epidemiology of low back pain. Best Pract Res Clin Rheumatol. 2010;24(6):769-81.

3. Betsch M, Schneppendahl J, Dor L, Jungbluth P, Grassmann JP, Windolf J, et al. Influence of foot positions on the spine and pelvis. Arthritis Care Res. 2011;63(12):1758-65.

4. Cibulka MT. Low back pain and its relation to the hip and foot. J Orthop Sports Phys Ther. 1999;29(10):595-601.

5. Menz HB, Dufour AB, Riskowski JL, Hillstrom HJ, Hannan MT. Foot posture, foot function and low back pain: the Framingham Foot Study. Rheumatol Oxf Engl. 2013;52(12):2275-82.

6. Brantingham JW, Lee Gilbert J, Shaik J, Globe G. Sagittal plane blockage of the foot, ankle and hallux and foot alignment-prevalence and association with low back pain. J Chiropr Med. 2006;5(4):123-7.

7. Kosashvili Y, Fridman T, Backstein D, Safir O, Bar Ziv Y. The correlation between pes planus and anterior knee or intermittent low back pain. Foot Ankle Int. 2008;29(9):910-3.

8. Brantingham JW, Adams KJ, Cooley JR, Globe D, Globe G. A single-blind pilot study to determine risk and association between navicular drop, calcaneal eversion, and low back pain. J Manipulative

Physiol Ther. June 2007;30(5):380-5.

9. Ogon M, Aleksiev AR, Pope MH, Wimmer C, Saltzman CL. Does arch height affect impact loading at the lower back level in running? Foot Ankle Int. 1999;20(4):263-6.

10. Khamis S, Yizhar Z. Effect of feet hyperpronation on pelvic alignment in a standing position. Gait Posture. 2007;25(1):127-34.

11. Pinto RZA, Souza TR, Trede RG, Kirkwood RN, Figueiredo EM, Fonseca ST. Bilateral and unilateral increases in calcaneal eversion affect pelvic alignment in standing position. Man Ther. 2008;13(6):513-9.

12. Bird AR, Bendrups AP, Payne CB. The effect of foot wedging on electromyographic activity in the erector spinae and gluteus medius muscles during walking. Gait Posture. 2003;18(2):81-91.

13. Castro-Méndez A, Munuera PV, Albornoz-Cabello M. The short-term effect of custom-made foot orthoses in subjects with excessive foot pronation and lower back pain: a randomized, double-blinded, clinical trial. Prosthet Orthot Int. 2013;37(5):384-90.

14. Mills K, Blanch P, Chapman AR, McPoil TG, Vicenzino B. Foot orthoses and gait: a systematic review and meta-analysis of literature pertaining to potential mechanisms. Br J Sports Med. 2010;44(14):1035-46.

15. Coste J, Le Parc JM, Berge E, Delecoeuillerie G, Paolaggi JB. French validation of a disability rating scale for the evaluation of low back pain (EIFEL questionnaire). Rev Rhum Ed Francaise 1993. 1993;60(5):335-41.

16. Chou MC, Huang JY, Hung YM, Perng WT, Chang R, Wei JCC. Flat foot and spinal degeneration: Evidence from nationwide population-based cohort study. J Formos Med Assoc Taiwan Yi Zhi. 2021;120(10):1897-906.

17. Dionne CE, Dunn KM, Croft PR, Nachemson AL, Buchbinder R, Walker BF, et al. A consensus approach toward the standardization of back pain definitions for use in prevalence studies. Spine. 2008;33(1):95-103.

18. Shabat S, Gefen T, Nyska M, Folman Y, Gepstein R. The effect of insoles on the incidence and severity of low back pain among workers whose job involves long-distance walking. Eur Spine J. 2005;14(6):546-50.

19. van den Hoogen HJ, Koes BW, van Eijk JT, Bouter LM, Devillé W. On the course of low back pain in general practice: a one year follow up study. Ann Rheum Dis. 1998;57(1):13-9.

20. Corp N, Mansell G, Stynes S, Wynne-Jones G, Mors(I L, Hill JC, et al. Evidence- based treatment recommendations for neck and low back pain across Europe: A systematic review of guidelines. Eur J Pain Lond Engl. 2021;25(2):275-95.

21. Glémarec J, Varin S, Cozic C, Tanguy G, Volteau C, Montigny P, et al. Efficacy of local glucocorticoid after local anaesthetic in low back pain with lumbosacral transitional vertebra: A randomized placebo-controlled double-blind trial. Joint Bone Spine. 2018;85(3):359-63.

22. Thomas EN, Pers YM, Mercier G, Cambiere JP, Frasson N,

Ster F, et al. The importance of fear, beliefs, catastrophizing and kinesiophobia in chronic low back pain rehabilitation. Ann Phys Rehabil Med. 2010;53(1):3-14.

23. Calmels P, Queneau P, Hamonet C, Le Pen C, Maurel F, Lerouvreur C, et al. Effectiveness of a lumbar belt in subacute low back pain: an open, multicentric, and randomized clinical study. Spine. 2009;34(3):215-20.

24. Njeze NR, Ezeofor SN, Agwu-Umahi OR. Plain radiographs of lumbar spine in patients with low back pain. Arch Osteoporos. 2018;13(1):104.

25. van Tulder MW, Assendelft WJ, Koes BW, Bouter LM. Spinal radiographic findings and nonspecific low back pain. A systematic review of observational studies. Spine. 1997;22(4):427-34.

26. Goldcher A. 8 - Static foot. In: Goldcher A, editor. Podologie (Sixième Édition) [Internet]. Paris: Elsevier Masson; 2012 [cited 4 Aug 2022]. p. 113-45. Available from: https://www.sciencedirect.com/science/article/pii/B9782294714818000080

27. Dalibon P. Affections rheumatological of the pied. Actual Pharm. 2018;57(579):50-3.

28. Biga N. Clinical examination of the foot and instep. Data collection and construction of etiopathogenic chains. Rev Chir Orthopédique Traumatol. 2009;95(4, Supplement):47-54.

29. Nait Khachat A, Amrani N, Meftah S, Belhaj K, Tchonda S, Elamari S, et al. Plantar hypertension and the diabetic foot: the role of

podoscopic assessment and preventive devices. Médecine Mal Métaboliques. 2016;10(3):270-4.

30. Uhl JF, Chahim M, Allaert FA. Static foot disorders: a major risk factor for chronic venous disease? Phlebol J Venous Dis. 2012;27(1):13-8.

31. Rothbart BA, Estabrook L. Excessive pronation: a major biomechanical determinant in the development of chondromalacia and pelvic lists. J Manipulative Physiol Ther. 1988;11(5):373-9.

32. Botte RR. An interpretation of the pronation syndrome and foot types of patients with low back pain. J Am Podiatry Assoc. 1981;71(5):243-53.

33. Builder MA, Marr SJ. Case history of a patient with low back pain and cavus feet. J Am Podiatry Assoc. 1980;70(6):299-301.

34. Dananberg HJ, Guiliano M. Chronic low-back pain and its response to custom- made foot orthoses. J Am Podiatr Med Assoc. 1999;89(3):109-17.

35. Sadler S, Spink M, Cassidy S, Chuter V. Prefabricated foot orthoses compared to a placebo intervention for the treatment of chronic nonspecific low back pain: a study protocol for a randomised controlled trial. J Foot Ankle Res. 2018;11:56.

36. Larsen K, Weidich F, Leboeuf-Yde C. Can custom-made biomechanic shoe orthoses prevent problems in the back and lower extremities? A randomized, controlled intervention trial of 146 military conscripts. J Manipulative Physiol Ther. 2002;25(5):326-31.

37. Tooms RE, Griffin JW, Green S, Cagle K. Effect of viscoelastic insoles on pain. Orthopedics. 1987;10(8):1143-7.

38. Cambron JA, Duarte M, Dexheimer J, Solecki T. Shoe orthotics for the treatment of chronic low back pain: a randomized controlled pilot study. J Manipulative Physiol Ther. 2011;34(4):254-60.

39. Sung PS, Zipple JT, Andraka JM, Danial P. The kinetic and kinematic stability measures in healthy adult subjects with and without flat foot. The Foot. 2017;30:21-6.

Appendix 1 Template

Full name :

File No.:

Telephone:

Occupation :

Place of residence: rural urban

Age :

Sex :

History:

Sport: 1-Yes 2-No If yes which1- Amateur 2- Professional
Weight= Height= BMI=

COMMON LUMBAGO :

-From

-EVA Low back pain

-Spinal syndrome -Walking on spikes -Examination of the hips		Root syndrome Walking on heels
-Knee statics: valgum	Normo-axed	Genu varum Genu
-Neurological examination		

-Current treatment:

1-Anatalgesics (level I / II)

2-NSAIDs (.)

3-Myorelaxants

4-Antidepressants

5- Pregabalin

6-physical treatment

7-Epidural infiltrations

8-Acupuncture

Functional impact: EIFEL questionnaire= Lumbar spine x-ray :
-Normal

Disc diseasePosterior inter-apophyseal arthrosis

Narrow lumbar canalSpondylolisthesis Other

STATIC FOOT DISORDER :

History of talalgia or metatarsalgia: noyes Current foot complaints:
1/ Talalgia: Nonoui inferior/posterior unilateral/bilateral Hourly

2/ Metatarsalgia:

Not present unilateral/bilateral

Schedule 2/ Trophic disorders of the skin or nails: YesNo

Type Location 3/ Footwear difficulties: YesNo
4/ Wearing of safety shoes or parts of uniform: Yes No
Examination of the feet :

1/ Type: 1-Egyptian2-Square3-Greek

Overall appearance of the feet: 1-oedema, 2-haematoma, 3-inflammatory area 2/ Asymmetry of heat, sweating or hairiness: YesNo

3/ Hyperkeratosis (callus): 1-Yes2-No Seat 4/ Corns: 1-Yes2-No Location

5/ Onychodystrophies: 1- Yes2-No Seat 6/ Intertrigo: 1- Yes2-No Location

7/ Deformations: 1- Yes2-No

Type (Hallux valgus, hammer toe, claw toe, quintus varus, supra/infra-adductus)

Reducible deformations: 1- Yes2-No

8/ Presence of exquisite pain points: 1-Yes2-No Location

9/ Joint amplitudes (talocrural / subtalar / Chopart / Lisfranc / MTP): 1-limited2-not limited

10/ Neurological examination of the feet :

11/Vascular examination: 0- Normal 1-ocre dermatitis, 2-telangiectasias, 3-varices

12/Gait examination: 1-littering 2-leaning 3-stepping 4-spastic or pseudo-ebriated gait

13/Podoscope test :

Foot 1-Normal 2-Flat 3-Hollow Stage (if flat/hollow foot)
Angle between the axis of the leg and the heel (valgus/varus) = 1:1.

Appearance of the calcaneus and Achilles:

1-tumescence

2-nodosity

3-bursitis Protrusion of the medial tubercle of the navicular bone: 1-Yes2-No

14-Examination of the shoe :

Heel height in cm=

Shoe fastening system=

Presence of areas of sole wear: YesNo Presence of areas of heel wear:YesNo Examination of foot orthoses if present:

Functional Incapacity Scale for the Evaluation of Low Back Pain (EIFEL)

Assessment :Initial D Intermediate D Final D DATE:

Socio-administrative information:

Last name

First name

We would like to know how your lower back pain affects your ability to carry out the activities of daily living.

If you are bedridden with back pain, tick this box and call it a day:

However, if you can stand up and remain standing for at least a few moments, answer the following questionnaire. You will be given a list of phrases. These sentences describe certain difficulties in carrying out a daily physical activity directly related to your lower back pain. Read each sentence carefully, keeping in mind the state you are in today because of your back pain. When you read a sentence that corresponds to a difficulty you are experiencing today, tick it off. If it doesn't, leave it blank and move on to the next sentence. Remember to tick only the sentences that apply to you today.

1	My back keeps me at home practically all the time	
2	I often change position to relieve the strain on my back	
3	I walk more slowly than usual because of my back	
4	Because of my back, I can't do any of the tasks I'm used to doing at home.	
5	Because of my back. I use the handrail to climb the stairs.	
6	Because of my back, I lie down more often to rest	
7	Because of my back, I have to use a support to get out of a wheelchair.	
8	Because of my back. I try to get others to do things for me.	
9	Because of my back, I dress more slowly than usual.	
10	I only stand for short periods because of my back.	
11	Because of my back, I try not to bend down or kneel down	
12	My back makes it hard for me to get up from a chair	
13	My back hurts most of the time	
14	My back makes it hard for me to turn over in bed	
15	I have less appetite because of my back pain	
16	Because of my back pain, I find it hard to put on my socks (or stockings or tights).	
17	I can only walk short distances because of my back pain	
18	I'm sleeping less because of my back pain	
19	Because of my back, someone helps me get dressed	
20	Because of my back, I sit down most of the day	
21	Because of my back, I avoid doing major work around the house	
22	Because of my back pain, I'm more irritable than usual and in a bad mood with people.	
23	Because of my back, I climb the stairs more slowly than usual	
24	My back keeps me in bed most of the time	

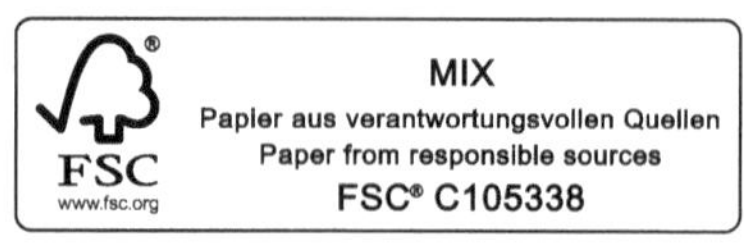

Printed by Books on Demand GmbH, Norderstedt / Germany